MW01595000

The Pocket Guide to Nursing in Corrections

How to succeed in any correctional environment

Volume 1

Author

Anneika EL-Houti

The Pocket Guide to Nursing in Corrections

Copyright © 2010
Anneika El-Houti

All Rights Reserved

Introduction

I can't tell you how many times I have been asked, "Why do you work in a Jail?" They would say, "I would be so scared around all those criminals!" The first time I was asked that question my thought process was a little different. I applied for the job as a way to help contribute to my household when I knew that the contract from the military duty was ending. I wanted to be in Law Enforcement like my husband. At the end of the day, we both wanted to feel like we were contributing to our community. There was a problem........ He did not want me to apply if I did get the job, he thought I would get into a fight and quit. So when I applied to work in the local correctional facility it was not as a nurse, I was as a deputy. I went for the first interview which was the walk through. The inmates were just as I imagined them to be. Some were respectful, but majority of the others were as vulgar as they could be. That alone told me whether I wanted to be there or not. The more I walked with the interviewer and the metal doors would slam shut as loud as prison doors could sound I felt the adrenaline rising inside of me. You will either feel a sense of seclusion or a sense of inner strength. I felt like if I got this job I could not let it beat me, not the doors slamming, the vulgar inmates or anything else. I will win and most of all, my husband will not get the satisfaction of saying that he told me so. I felt in my heart that even though they are incarcerated for a reason, my purpose was not to further condemn them. It was to ensure their safety as well as that of the community and to make sure all the deputies (including myself) and the non-security working staff got home safely. I felt at first that I was just doing my job. The pay was better than any full time civilian job I had ever had and it was rather a think less job so I thought. The more I worked and the more I went to church and allowed God to minister to me. I found that I became more aware of the lost souls that were in these institutions, deputies and inmates alike. I felt like there had to be more to this than just a job. My Bishop always spoke about striving for excellence in every aspect of your life. So one day I woke in the morning and asked God, "What will you have me do today

Lord?" His response to me was to listen. So for the next year or so that is what I did. I heard all kinds of sad, victorious and controversial stories from inmates as well as deputies. Some I will take to my grave. In every instance I always asked God to tell me what he wanted me to say to them to offer comfort or inspiration or to minister. As God being as mighty and awesome as he has always been to me his words he gave to me were always perfect and appropriate. I did everything I could to be obedient and give the words he gave me, (not saying I gave it all the time due to my personal lack of trust in his divine order of things.) and for that I will eternally be grateful.

Acknowledgments

I want acknowledge my two mothers Linda El-Houti and Ollie West. Linda for giving life to me and pouring into me all that she could give to me of herself. My Bishop Daniel Robertson Jr. would say, "Some things are taught and some things are caught." I did not really under-stand that until my mother passed away. It was like God allowed the doors of wisdom to open my eyes. I want to acknowledge Ollie my aunt, for being obedient when God spoke to care for me when my mother could or did not want to. To my children Angelo, Marcellous and

Yazmen I just want to say thank you for being you. This book is to honor God for whom all blessings flow and to thank all those that took the time to render their talents to help me pass on God's message to love your neighbor as yourself. I hope this book will offer a little insight of what it is to be a nurse in corrections and how to succeed in this field. You can do it! And To God be the glory.

First Fear

Before you become a successful nurse
working in corrections you must first be
able to conquer your fear of the
correctional institutions. I'm not saying to
be fearless because you must have a
healthy fear of what and who you are
dealing with so that you can do a proper
assessment of how you can excel in your
environment. You must ask yourself a few
questions:

1. Can I care for a person that has killed or raped a child without thinking of what they did the entire time?

2. Can I be prompt in caring for an inmate that you know has committed a heinous crime and he/she feels like you owe them the pamper treatment?

3. Can you maintain professionalism when you have been called everything but a child of God, and still give the best treatment you know and have been trained to give?

4. Can you care for someone after you have been spat on?

5. Can you offer some bit of encouragement to a per-son who knows he will never see the light of day and knows

*why but they are still afraid to
die incarcerated?*

*I know these are some very hard questions to
answer but these are real questions. These
are situations you may have to face at some
point in your journey in the correctional
nursing field. You must understand why you
are there and know what you are there to
do. Once you have gotten passed that point
you must go through the next personal
check- up, the initial walk through during
your interview. If you have never worked in
any type of correctional setting, I promise
you it is not a cakewalk but it is doable.
Please understand that as you are gaining*

information and mentally filtering your environment (the jail, or prison) the interviewer and the inmates are sizing you up. You must look confident even if inside you want to run for the door. It is a natural fight or flight reaction you cannot avoid. Make sure you look at every aspect of the facility. How do the inmates move throughout the facility? Are they in well secured areas or do you see them securing themselves? Do the deputies greet you or they or do they only speak because the Interviewer introduced you to the? Does it look like the facility is clean or does it smell like stinky, sweaty body odor? Are the floors

cleans? Are the deputies looking at you like

you're lunch, just like the inmates or are they

respectful? Do you even meet any deputies?

What does your gut tell you? Once you get

home sit and replay it all in your mind

because what you see is the best of the best.

Reality will start on day two. The first week

of work will definitely tell you whether you

are fit for the job or if this is not your cup of

tea. Every day the inmates will make it their

business to try and find out as much

information about you by what you tell them

in the questions they ask or the questions

you don't answer. The best way to deal with the barrage of questions is to tell them what you want them to know that is allowed by security. Tell them frankly, "That is none of your business." Most inmates know that they have limits. They just want to know what your limits with them are. You should be scheduled for a security class on such things as what not to bring into the jail and what not to do in front of the inmates. Pay very close attention this class is given for a reason. Don't go in-to the jail with the mentality that all inmates are horrible people. Some or most of them are people just like you and I who have made a bad

decision and now have to pay for it. They just

want to do their time and go home. You

must not use their charge as a reason to

either treat them or allow them to suffer. At

the same time you may be faced with caring

for a man/woman that has committed a

horrendous crime and are in dire need of

care that you may have to give. It is always

safer to lean on the side of precaution and

use your policy and procedure to the letter as

well as making no movement to care without

the security officer. ***Example: It was the first***

day of orientation for Nurse Judy at the

county jail. Prior to working at the jail she had worked for a year at The Willow Palace Nursing home. She was used to 60 beds of elderly people who relied on management of their care along with two CAN workers. For the most part the work was heavy as far as documenting, but task wise it was fairly easy, as long as the CNA did their jobs her work was a cakewalk. Worst -case scenario she had to assist in the care of the patients and had to deal with the family telling her how they did/did not like the way she responded to their family member's care. She had a very short class that gave her a brief idea on what she will see, but when the security officer walks her upstairs for her tour of where she is going to work she had no idea what to expect.

Once she walked on the floor she is wearing fitting jeans (A no, no anyway for a first day!) and the inmates go into a frenzy. Some of these inmates had not seen a woman, that close up, that was behind a window. They try to ask her a thousand questions at once.

"Whatz your name?

How old are you?

Are you single?

When are you starting work here?

Where you from?

Can I have some of that?

The questions began to become more and more derogatory and more and more vulgar. By the time she walked off that floor her face was so red from embarrassment, and needless to say she never came back. Could that have been avoided? I think so, if she knew what to expect.

My Presentation

Just when you thought you were done presenting yourself once you were offered the job. That was just the beginning. You now have to present yourself as a reliable, trustworthy extension to the inmate as well as the security officer. Here is the reason why: before you ever thought about working for any corrections department has had a number of nurses that have created havoc by having inappropriate relationships with in-mates and bringing in things that they knew were not allowed to be brought in, They came *in and were either not mentally prepared for the job and left after day one, or treated the in- mates so horribly that they were asked to leave or walked out of the facility. So now here comes you and they all, including your co-workers, want to see how you will stand up. Will you come to work with your uniform so tight that the inmates only want you to care for them? Will you tell the inmate, "That's why your #4^$% is in jail and I am going home!" or will you be the nurse that takes pride in her work, tries to be on time every day, keeping your personal comments to yourself about co-workers unless it directed* to that co-worker? Don't make it a habit to tell all your business to every-one that will listen. This will cause your co-workers to avoid you if they are no longer interested in you crying on everyone's shoulder. Every day make it your business to look neat, clean, and maintain your professionalism. If you tell your co- worker or supervisor that you are going to does something make sure you do it. Once you have destroyed that trust between you and your co- worker or supervisor then it will cause a great difficulty in them believing that you are a man/woman of your word if you have proven to them that you are not reliable.

It is also very important to do whatever it is you say you are going to do. If you tell an inmate you are going to check into something for him/her make sure you do that. A lot of inmates have a great deal of lack of trust in the correctional system because a lot of correctional professionals don't find the inmate important enough to keep their word for whatever reason. Don't be surprised that when you say you will check on something they may ask five other people to remind you to do the task or ask five other people to do what they asked you to do. They just want the job done. Once you have established a sense of trust you won't have to worry about them asking you more than one time about taking care of something. On that same note if you don't do what you say you will do with the security officer it takes away from your integrity with them. Sooner or later it will be your word against theirs and they won't stand by you if they feel you lied to them and did not do what you said you would do. So if you can't do it, just tell them that you will try and make an effort.

Example: Nurse Jane: I told inmate Jenkins that I would look in his chart for an order for him to have a special tray.

Can you pull his chart if you're going to the record room? Nurse Linda: I told him I would do that yesterday, you are such a good nurse. I ain't got time to look for some stupid chart for a special tray order! He wasn't thinking about some special tray on the street, but I'll pull it for you. This is why inmates will ask more than one person to have the one task accomplished. This may be one reason why an inmate/security officer has a lack of trust in the medical department. You can make the difference by being the one nurse out of many nurses that make it their business

to complete what they start and to do

whatever it is was said to be done. It not

only builds confidence in you as a nurse,

but it allows the inmate and other staff

the sense of respect and trust in you for

being a man or woman of your word.

Document, Document, Document

This can either make you or break you. It can

be the determining factor that defines you as

a nurse. A very wise Director of Nursing gave

me this advice and it brought me right back

to nursing school where I found that I could

administer care for strangers without fear of

personal ridicule was. If you don't document

what happened, it didn't happen." What that

means is, if you did a proper assessment on

the inmate and reported your findings to the

doctor, went home at the end of your shift,

reported back to work the next day to find

that the inmate had passed and you forgot

to place a detailed nurse's note on what you did and what you reported to the doctor in the inmate's chart, What you did never happened and the doctor could easily say you never told him/her anything. During the investigation by Internal Affairs, the inmate's Lawyer, and your supervisor, as well as possible the nursing board you will have the weight to bear on your own about what really happened. It is your word against the doctor, other eye witnesses, and anyone else who saw what really happened, all because you did not document it when it happened. It is very important that with everything you *do there is a paper trail, or computer log note to support it. From giving an inmate's medication to a conversation you had with an inmate on him/her feeling depressed. These fine and sometime daunting details can make you as a nurse. The reason for that is if you are diligent in your documenting there is no question in what you have done during your shift and that will carry over to your work ethic by taking this time. Some things to be careful to put in your notes are: Time, date, what happened, what the inmate said was wrong, what makes it worse or better, what you did, and what the plan of action was after. Last but not least, what*

was reported to the doctor, how did you

report? (By phone, in person, or via email),

what did he tell you to do? All these things

play a role in the bigger picture of how the

care for the inmate was conducted during

his/her stay in your facility. You can be the

difference in whether they get standard care

or exceptional care within the confines of the

protocols of your facility. By maintaining

good notes it holds the responsible parties

accountable to what happened last and

alleviates you from being implicated as that

nurse that did not follow up or be subject to

the accusation of neglecting to following

through. This can be considered cruel and

unusual punishment. Now the flip side; if

you as a nurse not familiar with

documenting everything that you do or tend

to have memory lapses, (senior moments)

then carry a note pad with you. It can be a

small note pad that can fit in your pocket

and when something happens just jot down

the date, time, name of the person involved,

as well as vital signs if it is an emergency

response, all these things are key for when

the situation calms down you have accurate

information to document with. If there was

more than one person responding to an

emergency situation you may want to put

down the deputies that responded with you

by name. That can also be very helpful. With

saying that it is very important to know your

policy and procedure, not just from the

stand- point of the facility you work, but also

from the perspective of the company you

work for and what they require from you. It

could be very disheartening if you find out

you were fired due to being out of

compliance with your company policy and

you did not know. The company will not

always make you aware of what their policy

is until you mess up and they will ask you,

"Didn't you read your handbook we gave you

that you signed to say you understood?"

Whether you say yes or no does not really

matter; they assume you are liable because

they won't be. It is in your best interest to

protect yourself and document details and

events as they happen. Here is one bonus

tidbit of advice to be aware of as well. Make

sure if you are working with someone as a

team, be so very sure to check and double

check that their part is done before signing

your name. In the end, if you are ultimately

responsible for signing off and the other

person part is not done then the task is

incomplete and I promise you; you will take

all of the responsibility for it not being done

in its entirety.

Making Friends

In this type of environment it is so important

for you to know that it is not necessary to

discussing your personal business around

inmates, you would think that correctional

officers, deputies and medical professionals

really take heed. It is important that you

know when you work for a new job not to

think that you will make or find your new

best friend. That is not what you are there

for and often times you will find yourself with

hurt feelings by the person you thought you

could trust. I am not saying that long time

friendships don't develop in work settings.

However, if you go to work looking for just

that, chances are you may become a victim

of rumor. In any work setting there are

people who are natural nurturers. These

people are good trainers because that does

not mean you can trust your personal

business with them. You must be able to do

your job and do it well during your time on

the clock. Once off the clock you can do as

you please, but be aware that what you do

off the clock can also affect your job.

Example: Nurse Omar went out with Officer Michelle over the weekend, but Officer Danna likes Nurse Omar. When they all came back to work Officer Danna makes a comment about what she heard happened over the weekend and Officer Michelle responds back and they have a verbal altercation. Nurse Omar and all involved were dismissed because he did not adhere to the no fraternization Policy and by not adhering caused problems.

From the time you start work until the time

you leave the job you should want to have healthy working relationships. It is imperative be able to tell when a work related association has become toxic and allow the association with that person to pass without grudges or animosity. I promise you in the medical field you will see them or work with them again. They may be your supervisor. Professionalism is the most important thing you need to remember when dealing with other professionals. Don't allow your emotions write a check you cannot cash. Meaning, it doesn't allow you to be angry right now and say or do something that may negatively affect you in *the future. Now if/when you make a lifelong friend, if a new friendship evolves with another person, don't treat the new person like an outsider because they are not like you and your friend. Don't shut them out when the new person starts; you should remember what it felt like when you started. Exhibiting this behavior means you have formed a "clique." Cliques are counterproductive in any work environment, especially when the goal is to ostracize any new person. It can cause a hostile work environment. This will be discussed later in the next chapter.*

Avoiding the "Cliques"

We all know what the word clique means.

When you were in school and there were

always different groups, **the popular ones,**

the Athletes, the Academic groups and so

on. You could always tell who they were

and who they associated with by who they

talked or did not talk to, who they spent

time with during school hours and what

they said they did with each other after

school hours. They did not have to accept

anyone that was not like them; in fact they

usually made a point of rejecting those

that were not like them. You will run into

the same in the work place. The difference

is you don't have to fit anywhere or with

any particular group. Some groups will

make you think if you don't join it will

affect your career, which only makes a

difference if you are in a union. That is a

positive group in place to protect your

rights. That's not a clique. What I am

referring to is when you go to work on a

different shift due to shortage and a

particular group of nurses are used to

working with their set of people where

they take two hour lunches and cover for

each other and make a great deal of

personal phone calls, and try their best to

do as little work as possible during shift.

When you come to help you become a

threat. So you don't feel encouraged to

take the shift again while you're there they

whisper around you, order lunch and not

ask you and eat together while you're

there. They may bring in special treats like

cookies and say, "I bought them for you

cause I know how much you like them," but

never ask you whether you want any while

they eat them. This behavior is not only

condescending and immature, but it

ostracizes the nurse who is working to help

the shift and it is a breeding ground for a

hostile environment. As a new employee

the strain of being a new employee in a

new work environment paired with feeling

like you cannot approach your co-workers

can be a deciding factor on whether or not

your company will retain the new nurse. As

a supervisor it can be disheartening and

difficult to discourage this behavior. If a

supervisor is a proficient as they should be

they already know who they are, but are

either part of it or has turned a blind eye to

it due to the effectiveness of the work

results of these particular employees. The

one way you as a nurse can do your part in

dealing with the behavior is to know who

you are and what you have accomplished

as a professional. Work on becoming

comfortable in your own professional skin

and in your new work environment and try

not to take offense to what you may

experience as a result of the cli-ques.

Focus on why you are there and not who

you are there with. It is important that you

understand that this is a profession in

which you may and will cross paths again

so making enemies is not beneficial but at

the same time you don't have to be a

doormat. You want to always maintain

professionalism while you're working with

your co-workers and at the same time re-

member to treat each person as an

individual and not hold one person

responsible for the actions of a few; some

people are natural followers just like it was

in high school. If this message is talking

about you then you need to remember

when you started your first day of work.

How was the staff to you? Did they make

you feel welcome? Did you feel like you

could ask them anything or did they make

you feel inadequate for asking? Don't get

me wrong it is very good that you have

friends that you work with, but understand

that there is a time and a place for

everything. And your best friend forever

(BFF) can be that as long as it does not

offend other co-workers and disrupt the

flow of the work environment. Take all the

feelings and emotions you felt the first

week of work, good, bad and take the good

and duplicate it and try and make sure the

bad is not repeated for the next person.

These are the makings of a leader. If it

becomes a problem to where you as the

new nurse find it difficult to come to work

due to the way you are being treated, talk

to someone before deciding to leave the

job. It may be a resolvable situation.

Fraternization

Every company has a policy on fraternization. It is important that you know these policies prior to looking for your "Boaz" in the correctional facility. Some facilities' rules are stricter than others, but you need to know them. Let's explain what fraternization really is: it could be a medical professional who has a relationship with an in- mate that they may not have known prior to their incarceration. It could be a medical professional who is dating another staff

member in the same facility. It could be a

person obtaining a job in a correctional

facility for the purpose of being closer to

someone they are dating or married to

without the knowledge of the

administration. Whatever the case may be

fraternization is something that should be

handled with care. It can be the difference

between your professional success and

professional suicide. I picked this time to talk

about this subject because once you are able

to have all the things in place in the previous

chapter you can become comfortable and

whether you are married or not it is easy to

let your guard down and make a big mistake

that can destroy your career. Let me give you

an example:

Nurse Joan started working at a the

jail and rumors have started that she is

showing special attention to Inmate John

as well as being seen by deputies

spending one on one time due to the

inmate being called out for a Sick Call visit

by her. It was reported to the Director of

Nursing (DON) and when asked about it she denied all accusations. After six months she quits. Four months later Nurse Joan submits a request to be married to inmate John.

Now what she did will cause questions to come in the mind of administrators on what are the intentions of any other nurse? Will they smuggle in contraband to please the inmate? The trust factor is greatly jeopardized.

Here is another example: Nurse Frank and Deputy Linda have been seen having lunch together in the break room for about a month. No one thinks anything of it because it is their time and business.

Six months later,

Deputy Linda is five months pregnant. Again no one's business, the problem now is people are asking Nurse Frank is he the reason for her pregnancy and he is denying it and it gets back to Deputy Linda. She then causes a scene and threatens to take him to court as well as make his job a living Hell!

Any of these situations can happen outside of the correctional facility. The difference is it did not. The Sheriff or Warden has to

make the work environment safe for both

the public as well as the inmate. The rules

were put in place for a reason. Both

situations are a compromise of security and

a hard hit on the person's professional

behavior but it can be avoided. Don't make

a habit of dating where you work, but if you

do date where you work keep it out of the

work place. The less you offer of your

personal business the less of a security risk

you become to the facility.

Be Smart

When you work in the medical profession,

you are hired based on your experience,

knowledge and your ability to be fit to work

in this type of environment. Once you start it

is in your best interest to become the best at

your job for as long as you are there. You

don't have to lower your moral standards to

be promoted or allow yourself to become a

doormat for anyone to excel in your job.

Make it your job to become an asset to the

company. They will appreciate and it this will

allow you to ask for some things and not feel

any obligation because you have earned it. If

you make it your motivation every day that

when you see a need, you fill a need if it is

within your ability, you will be successful.

With that being said it is also important you

manage your money well. This profession

can pay very well and it can pay very poorly,

depending on where you live and how much

time you have under your belt. If you don't

really know how to manage money get some

counseling. You can go from making fifteen

dollars an hour to twenty dollars an hour

depending on the position and if you don't

know how to manage your finances if your

pay ever changes you will be financially devastated. It is imperative you carry outside life insurance from what your job offers that will cover you if you ever leave your job. Make short term and long term goal for your career as well as your finances. The Word states in Hosea 4: 6 (KJV)

"*My people perish from a lack of knowledge.*"

If you didn't know then you would surely perish, well now you know so be prosperous and be a blessing to someone else as I pray this book is to you.

*** *Here are a few tips for your journey****

It is imperative you carry outside life

insurance from what your job offers that

will cover you if you ever leave your job.

Make short term and long term goals for

your career as well as your finances.

For example: In 6 months I want to have

$500 dollars in my savings account. I want

to have my RN by 2012 or if you have your

RN choose an educational goal. It is

important that you have goals, write

them down, date them, and mark them

off when you have obtained them along

with a date. Allowing yourself to have

goals and see those being obtained allows

you to feel accomplished and empowered.

Word to the Wise

Working in Corrections it does require

you is not a hard job, but know the

do's and don'ts. It can be a very

fulfilling job if you want to give back

to your community, and it pays well.

You also have the opportunity to learn

acute care, quick but thorough

assessments, and detailed

documenting. This is a career that has

its challenges like any other but it is

well worth the effort. I have worked in

this field enough to know that I love it

and you will find that you either love it

or hate it. You will determine that on

your own and it won't take long. Don't

give up before you start because you

see the rigid exterior of the facility.

Walk through and explore it. You will

find that you become more alert to

your environment and you will see

people far past what they have done

and learn to view them for who they

are or who they show you and that is

ok. The bottom line is that at the end

of the day you go home with a sense

of accomplishment and you want that

opportunity to do it again the next

day. I hope I was able to give you a

glimpse of what it is like to be a nurse

in the correctional field and maybe

spark an interest in this wonderful

field. See you there. God Bless.

About the Author

I am a single mother of four   Angelo, Marcellous, and beautiful gifts from God Tamira, Yazmen. I now reside in Virginia where I work as a Correctional Nurse. I have worked in corrections for over seven years now. I began writing when I was elementary school as a stress reliever. It was a way I could express what I felt without getting in trouble for being rude. I was very interested in poetry and found that to be my outlet. Combining my love for God and my desire to see his glory is acknowledged allowed this short rendition to flow from me. I hope this

book blesses you as it blessed me to put on

paper.

Made in the USA
Columbia, SC
02 May 2022

59805251R00037